The Plant-Based Diet for Beginners

The Health Benefits of Eating a Plant-Based Diet.

21-Day Meal Plan, Shopping List and Easy Recipes That Will Make You Drool

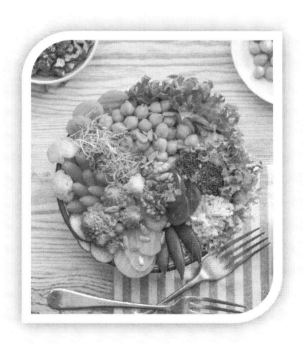

D1524495

Alice Newman © 2020

Table of Contents

INTRODUCTION

You may have already heard about the plant-based diet, but you may not know precisely what it is. In this chapter, you'll learn precisely what the plant-based diet is and how it can help you. First, let's take a look at whole foods. Whole foods are unprocessed foods. A plant-based diet concentrates on whole food. Whole foods include whole bread, whole wheat pasta, nondairy milk, nuts, seed butter, and tofu. Of course, you can also eat herbs and spices, nuts and seeds, fruits and vegetables, and legumes such as lentils and beans. All of these will make a diet based on plants.

Many people mistake the plant-based diet for a vegan one. So, let's talk about the difference. There are parallels in both of them, but there are small differences. A vegan diet does not include any products based on animals. This, of course, contains meats but also eggs and outcomes of these animals, such as honey. Vegans will carry this perspective into their life as well, which is more than a diet to them. A plant-based diet will keep you from eating anything based on animals, but it will not prevent you from using animal products in your life.

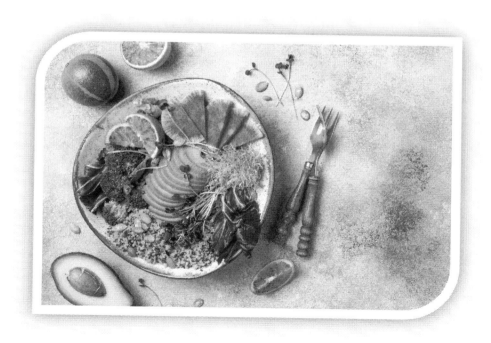

THE BENEFITS

Now that you know what the plant-based diet is, it's essential to look at the host of benefits that it has to offer. It's hard to stick to a diet that makes you drastically change your current way of eating if you don't have a good reason. That's what this chapter is about. Giving you that good reason to meet your health and weight loss goals using the plant-based diet.

LOWERS BLOOD PRESSURE

A plant-based diet has been proven to lower blood pressure because it has a high potassium content. A plant-based diet reduces blood pressure as well as stress and anxiety. Potassium-rich foods include seeds, whole, almonds, beans, berries, and grain. However, meat contains almost no potassium, which is why the plant-based diet offers a better way to control your blood pressure.

LOWERS CHOLESTEROL

Plants don't contain cholesterol, which includes saturated forms such as coffee or chocolate. When you live a plant-based diet lifestyle, you're reducing the amount of cholesterol you take in to next to zero. A plant-based diet will lower your risk of heart disease since cholesterol is a leading cause of stroke and heart attack.

MAINTAINS BLOOD SUGAR LEVELS

The plant-based diet has a lot of protein. Protein can lower blood sugar production, and in turn, it will leave you feeling full for longer. Also, a plant-based diet can help to reduce stress levels by lowering the cortisone levels in the body. Cortisol is a stress hormone.

STAVES OFF CHRONIC DISEASE

Chronic diseases, including diabetes, cancer, and obesity, are low in societies that follow a plant-based lifestyle. This diet has been proven to help to fight off chronic disease by helping to reduce chronic inflammation, high blood sugar, stress, and provides your body with the nutrients it needs.

WEIGHT LOSS

In societies that follow a mainly plant-based lifestyle, obesity is also lower, which we've already covered as a chronic disease. Since you're taking in more vitamins and nutrients as well as fiber, which your body has to break down. While you're eating a plant-based lifestyle, you're also likely to stay fuller for longer, which means you'll eat less overall. To lose weight, you have to burn more calories than you take in, so eating less is an essential part of that.

MORE ENERGY

Within days of this type of eating, you'll feel energized because you'll get the nutrients you need. The foods that you'll be eating will also have higher water content, which can hydrate your skin and leave you feeling better overall. Plant-based foods are easier to digest and lighter, so you'll feel better than ever in just a few days. You'll also get a better sleep when you eat right. When you feed your body the vitamins and

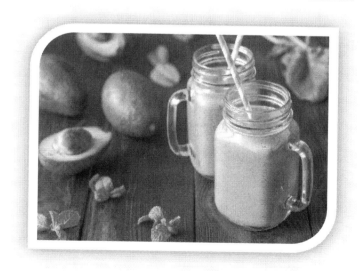

minerals it needs, you'll help your body relax and give it a peaceful sleep. Calcium and magnesium can help to relax the body for quiet rest, which this diet is packed full of.

BASIC SHOPPING LIST

While this shopping list does not include everything for original recipes, this shopping list will help you to keep your pantry stocked with the basics.

VEGETABLES: NON-STARCHY

These vegetables are excellent for your body because they are packed with nutrients and will help to get you the vitamins you need. This includes your leafy greens such as kale, spinach, butter lettuce, etc. You can also use eggplant, zucchini, tomatoes, and brocco li as your non-starchy basics.

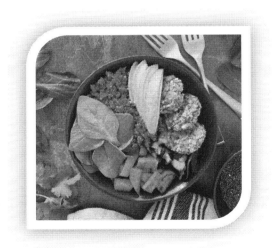

VEGETABLES: STARCHY

This includes all types of potatoes, whole corn, legumes of all kinds. This consists of all beans and lentils, root vegetables, and even quinoa. These are filling parts of your meals, which are packed with fiber.

WHOLE GRAINS

You need some sort of grain in your plant-based diet. Whole grains are always recommended, including whole wheat, brown rice, and oats. Over processed oats will not give you the nutrients you need.

FRUITS

Any whole fruits are available on the plant-based diet. However, it is recommended that you avoid dried fruits and juiced fruits because of the sheer amount of sugar it'll pack into your diet.

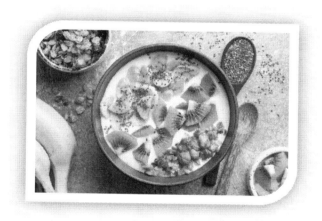

BEVERAGES

You can have almost any drinks on your plant-based diet. However, it's recommended that you drink unsweetened plant-based kinds of milk, decaffeinated tea, decaffeinated coffee, and green tea.

SPICES

As far as spices are concerned, any spices are allowed. This includes dried spices and fresh herbs.

OMEGA 3 SOURCES

With an all plant-based diet, you'll need omega three sources. These include ground flax seed as well as chia seeds.

NUTS

Any nuts are recommended on the plant-based diet, but it's useful to have peanuts and walnuts on hand. You can also keep cashews and almonds since they are used regularly in different dishes.

CONSUME SPARINGLY

These are plant-based foods, but they aren't as healthy for you as other plants. So, while you can have them, it's recommended that you use these sparingly. This includes added sweeteners. Examples of added sweeteners are fruit juice concentrate, natural sugars, honey, and maple syrup. Pumpkin seeds, sesame seeds, sunflower seeds, and dried fruits should also be consumed on a limited basis. Coconuts and avocados as well. You should also limit your refined wheat protein or soy protein

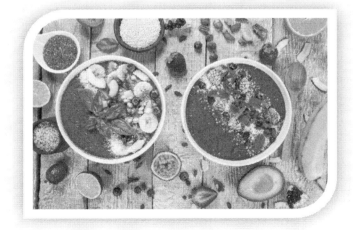

21 DAY MEAL PLAN

In this chapter, we'll go over a twenty-one-day meal plan with all of the recipes right in this book! By having a meal plan for a few weeks when you start a new diet, it's more likely that you'll stick to it.

DAY 1

Breakfast: Chia Banana Pudding

Lunch: Plant Pad Thai

Dinner: Tofu Bowl

DAY 2

Breakfast: Breakfast Polenta

Lunch: Collard Green Pasta

Dinner: Pad Thai Bowl

DAY 3

Breakfast: Green Banana Smoothie

Lunch: Eggplant Pasta

Dinner: Ginger Soba Noodle Bowl

DAY 4

Breakfast: Blue Zucchini Smoothie

Lunch: Tart Cabbage Soup

Dinner: Blackeye Pea Burritos

DAY 5

Breakfast: Spirulina Power Smoothie

Lunch: Parsnip & Matzo Soup

Dinner: Coconut Curry Noodles

DAY 6

Breakfast: Kicking Mango Smoothie

Lunch: Red Lentil Pasta

Dinner: Fung Tofu with Roasted Chickpeas

DAY 7

Breakfast: Chickpea Omelet

Lunch: Walnut & Orange Pasta

Dinner: Yellow Wild Rice Soup

DAY 8

Breakfast: Pumpkin Pie Oatmeal

Lunch: Cream of Broccoli Soup

Dinner: Sesame Stir Fry

DAY 9

Breakfast: Basic Kale Smoothie

Lunch: White Wine Pasta

Dinner: Sunday Roast

DAY 10

Breakfast: Breakfast Apple Bowl

Lunch: Quinoa Cranberry Salad

Dinner: Plant-Based Shepard's Pie

DAY 11

Breakfast: Overnight Chia Oats

Lunch: Pesto Quinoa

Dinner: Carrot & Turmeric Soup

DAY 12

Breakfast: Chia Banana Pudding

Lunch: Eggplant Pasta

Dinner: Bibimbap bowl

DAY 13

Breakfast: Chickpea Omelet

Lunch: Pesto Quinoa

Dinner: Mango Chickpea Curry with Plantain Chips

DAY 14

Breakfast: Green Banana Smoothie

Lunch: Tart Cabbage Soup

Dinner: Coconut Curry Noodles with Vegetable Satay

DAY 15

Breakfast: Kicking Mango Smoothie

Lunch: Vegetable Stir Fry

Dinner: Sesame Stir Fry

DAY 16

Breakfast: Breakfast Polenta

Lunch: Eggplant Pasta

Dinner: Stuffed Southwest Peppers

DAY 17

Breakfast: Golden Smoothie

Lunch: Kale & Quinoa Salad

Dinner: Wild Rice Lemon Soup

DAY 18

Breakfast: Spirulina Power Smoothie

Lunch: Walnut & Orange Pasta

Dinner: Blackeye Pea Burritos with Stuffed Portobello

DAY 19

Breakfast: Chickpea Omelet

Lunch: Collard Green Pasta

Dinner: Stuffed Southwest Peppers with Easy Collard Greens

DAY 20

Breakfast: Golden Smoothie

Lunch: Carrot & Chickpea Salad

Dinner: Sunday Roast

DAY 21

Breakfast: Breakfast Polenta

Lunch: Parsnip & Matzo Soup

Dinner: Sesame Stir Fry

BREAKFAST
RECIPES

PINK SMOOTHIE

Serves: 2

Time: 5 Minutes

Ingredients:

- 1 Cup Strawberries, Fresh
- 1 Cup Honey Melon
- 1 Cup Raspberries
- 1 Tablespoon Chia seeds
- ½ Cup Coconut Milk
- 1 Cup Water
- 2 Tablespoons Mint, Fresh & Chopped

Directions:

1. Blend everything until smooth.

BERRY MUESLI BOWL

Serves: 4

Time: 10 Minutes

Ingredients:

- 1 Cup Rolled Oats
- 1 Cup Quinoa
- 2 Cups Puffed Cereal
- ¼ Cup Sunflower Seeds
- ¼ Cup Raisins
- ¼ Cup Almonds
- ¼ Cup Cranberries, Dried
- ¼ Cup Figs, Dried
- ¼ Cup Coconut, Shredded & Unsweetened
- ¼ Cup Chocolate Chips, Non-Dairy
- 3 Teaspoons Cinnamon
- ½ Cup Coconut Milk
- ¾ Cup Muesli

Directions:

1. Mix everything and serve immediately.

CHIA BANANA PUDDING

Serves: 2

Time: 10 Minutes

Ingredients:

- ¼ Cup Chia Seeds
- ½ Cup Coconut Milk
- ½ Cup Almond Milk
- 1 Teaspoon Cinnamon
- 1 Tablespoon Agave
- 1 Banana, Mashed
- 1 Banana, Chopped
- Coconut Flakes to Taste

Directions:

1. Start by mixing your banana mash, almond milk, cinnamon, agave and chia seeds in a bowl with coconut milk. Cover the bowl and let it sit for at least an hour or overnight.
2. Garnish with coconut and bananas to serve.

OVERNIGHT CHIA OATS

Serves: 2

Time: 1 Hour 10 Minutes

Ingredients:

- ¾ Cup Rolled Oats
- ¼ Cup Almond Milk
- ½ Cup Water
- 1 Tablespoon Maple Syrup
- 1 Tablespoon Chia Seeds
- ¼ Teaspoon Ground Cinnamon
- ¼ Teaspoon Vanilla Extract, Pure
- Canned Blueberries to Garnish

Directions:

1. Mix all ingredients and then allow it to sit for an hour or overnight.
2. Stir the oats before garnishing with blackberries to serve.

PUMPKIN PIE OATMEAL

Serves: 4

Time: 35 Minutes

Ingredients:

- 3 Cups Almond Milk
- 1 Cup Steel Cut Oats
- 2 Tablespoons Maple Syrup
- 1 Cup Pumpkin Puree, Unsweetened
- 1/8 Teaspoon Ground Cloves
- ¼ Teaspoon Ground Nutmeg
- 1 Teaspoon Ground Cinnamon

Directions:

1. Get out a saucepan and bring your milk to a boil using medium-high heat. Reduce to low to simmer, adding in the pumpkin puree, oats, cinnamon, cloves, nutmeg, and maple syrup.
2. Cover, cooking for an additional half-hour. Stir every few minutes, and serve warm.

SCRAMBLED EGGS & MUSHROOMS

Serves: 6

Time: 50 Minutes

Ingredients:

- 1 Red Onion, Diced & Peeled
- 1 Red Bell Pepper, Seeded & Diced
- 1 Green Bell Pepper, Diced & Seeded
- 2 Cups Mushrooms, Fresh & Sliced
- 1 Head Cauliflower, Chopped into Florets
- Sea Salt & Black Pepper to Taste
- 1 ½ Teaspoons Turmeric
- ¼ Teaspoon Cayenne Pepper
- 2 Tablespoons Soy Sauce
- 3 Cloves Garlic, Minced & Peeled
- ¼ Cup Nutritional Yeast

Directions:

1. Place a skillet over medium heat, and toss in your peppers and mushrooms. Add the onions.
2. Cook for eight minutes, adding two tablespoons of water. Add the cauliflower in next, cooking for an additional six minutes.
3. Season with the remaining ingredients and cook for an additional five minutes before serving.

GOLDEN SMOOTHIE

Serves: 1

Time: 10 Minutes

Ingredients:

- 1/8 Teaspoon Black Pepper
- 1 Tablespoon Ginger, Fresh
- ½ Teaspoon Cinnamon
- ¼ Teaspoon Nutmeg, Ground
- ¼ Teaspoon Clove, Ground
- ¼ Cup Carrot Juice, Fresh
- 1 Cup Coconut Milk, Light
- 1 Cup Banana, Frozen, Ripe & Sliced
- 1 Tablespoon Hemp Seeds to Garnish

Directions:

1. Blend until smooth. Garnish with hemp seeds.

BREAKFAST APPLE BOWL

Serves: 2

Time: 10 Minutes

Ingredients:

- 2 Tablespoons Walnuts
- 1 Lemon, Juiced
- 6 Dates, Pitted
- 5 Apples
- ¼ Teaspoon Cinnamon, Ground

Directions:

1. Core the apples before dicing them. Leave them in large chunks.
2. Add the cinnamon, walnuts, dates, and lemon juice into a food processor before adding ¾ of your apples in too.
3. Blend and then serve topped with your remaining apples.

BLUE ZUCCHINI SMOOTHIE

Serves: 2

Time: 10 Minutes

Ingredients:

- ¼ Cup Greens
- 1 Banana, Frozen, Ripe & Sliced
- 1 Cup Blueberries
- 1 Stem Celery, Large
- 1 Tablespoon Hemp Seeds
- ¼ Teaspoon Cinnamon, Ground
- ½ Teaspoon Maca Powder
- 1 Cup Coconut Milk, Light

Directions:

1. Throw all ingredients into the blender, blending well before serving.

BREAKFAST POLENTA

Serves: 4

Time: 20 Minutes

Ingredients:

- 1 Teaspoon Cinnamon, Ground
- 1 Cup Polenta, Cooked
- 1 Cup Cranberries, Dried
- ¼ Cup Brown Rice Syrup
- 2 Pears, Cored, Diced & Peeled

Directions:

1. Place a saucepan over medium heat, and then heat your rice syrup. Toss in the pears and cranberries before sprinkling with cinnamon. Mix well, and cook for an additional ten minutes.
2. Serve over polenta.

GREEN BANANA SMOOTHIE

Serves: 2

Time: 10 Minutes

Ingredients:

- ½ Teaspoon Maca Powder
- ½ Cup Cucumber, Frozen
- 1 Tablespoon Hemp Seeds
- ½ Avocado, Ripe
- 1 Banana, Large, Peeled & Sliced
- 1 Scoop Protein Powder, Plain
- ½ Cup Greens
- ¾ Cup Almond Milk, Unsweetened

Directions:

1. Throw everything into your blender. Blend well until smooth.

CHICKPEA OMELET

Serves: 3

Time: 30 Minutes

Ingredients:

- ½ Teaspoon Baking Soda
- 1/3 Cup Nutritional Yeast
- 3 Green Onions, Chopped Roughly
- 4 Ounces Mushrooms, Sautéed
- Sea Salt & Black Pepper to Taste
- ½ Teaspoon Garlic Powder
- ½ Teaspoon Onion Powder
- 1 Cup Chickpea Flour

Directions:

1. Whisk the chickpea flour, onion powder, pepper, salt, garlic powder, baking soda, and yeast.
2. Stir a cup of water in, and blend into a batter.
3. Place a frying pan that is nonstick over medium heat. Put in a dollop over low heat, and cook with mushrooms and green onions. Flip the omelet and cook for another minute before serving.

KICKING MANGO SMOOTHIE

Serves: 2

Time: 10 Minutes

Ingredients:

- 2 ¼ Cup Mango, Frozen & Chopped
- 1 Cup Coconut Milk, Light
- 1 ¼ Cup Raspberries, Frozen
- 1 Lime, Juiced
- 1 Tablespoons Coconut, Shredded & Unsweetened
- 2 Tablespoons Ginger, Fresh
- 1/8 Teaspoon Cayenne Pepper
- 2 Tablespoons Hemp Seeds
- Coconut Yogurt to Serve
- Berries to Garnish
- Shredded Coconut to Garnish
- Hemp Seeds to Garnish

Directions:

1. Blend all ingredients except for your garnish. Make sure it's smooth, and garnish as desired.

SPIRULINA POWER SMOOTHIE

Serves: 1

Time: 20 Minutes

Ingredients:

- 1 Cup Baby Spinach
- 1 Teaspoon Spirulina Powder
- 1 Tablespoon Hemp Seed
- 1 Cup Coconut Milk, Light
- ½ Cup Cucumber, Sliced
- 1 Banana, Ripe
- ¼ Cup Granola for Garnish
- ¼ Cup Raspberries for Garnish

Directions:

1. Blend everything but your garnish. Once smooth garnish before serving chilled.

BASIC KALE SMOOTHIE

Serves: 2

Time: 10 Minutes

Ingredients:

- 1 Cup Mangos, Ripe, Cubed & Frozen
- 2 Cups Kale, Packed
- 1 Cup Ice
- 1 Cup Peaches, Frozen
- 1 Tablespoon Ginger, Fresh & Minced
- 1 Lemon, Juiced
- 1 Lime, Juiced
- 2 Cups Water
- 1 Tablespoon Maple Syrup, Raw

Directions:

1. Blend everything until smooth before serving chilled.

LUNCH RECIPES

COLLARD GREEN PASTA

Serves: 4

Time: 30 Minutes

Ingredients:

- 2 Tablespoons Olive Oil
- 4 Cloves Garlic, Minced
- 8 Ounces Whole Wheat Pasta
- ½ Cup Panko Bread Crumbs
- 1 Tablespoon Nutritional Yeast
- 1 Teaspoon Red Pepper Flakes
- 1 Large Lemon, Juiced & Zested
- 1 Bunch Collard Greens, Large

Directions:

1. Fill a pot with water and salt it. Bring it to a boil using high heat. Add in the pasta and cool al dente before rinsing under cold water to stop the cooking.
2. Reserve half a cup of the cooking liquid from the pasta and set it to the side.
3. Place it over medium heat and add in a tablespoon of olive oil. Stir in half of your garlic, sautéing for a half a minute.
4. Add in the breadcrumbs and then sauté, cooking for five more minutes.
5. Toss in the red pepper flakes and nutritional yeast, mixing well.
6. Transfer the breadcrumbs in the pan.
7. Add the remaining olive oil and then stir in your salt, pepper, garlic clove, and greens.
8. Cook for five minutes. Cook until wilted.
9. Add in the pasta, mix in the reserved pasta liquid, and then mix well. Add in the lemon juice, zest, and garlic crumbs. Toss before serving.

PLANT PAD THAI

Serves: 4

Time: 20 Minutes

Ingredients:

- 2 Teaspoons Coconut Oil
- 1 Red Pepper, Sliced
- 2 Carrots, Sliced
- ½ White Onion, Sliced
- 1 Thai Chili, Chopped
- 8 Ounces Brown Rice Noodles
- ½ Cup Peanuts, Chopped
- ½ Cup Cilantro, Chopped

Sauce:

- 3 Tablespoons Soy Sauce
- 3 Tablespoons Lime Juice, Fresh
- 3 Tablespoons Brown Sugar
- 1 Tablespoon Sriracha
- 3 Tablespoons Vegetable Broth
- 1 Teaspoon Chili Garlic Paste
- 2 Cloves Garlic, Minced

Tofu:

- 1 lb. Extra Firm Tofu, Sliced
- 1 Tablespoon Peanut Butter
- 2 Tablespoons Sriracha
- 3 Tablespoons Soy Sauce
- 2 Tablespoons Rice Vinegar

- 2 Teaspoons Sesame Oil
- 2 Teaspoons Ginger, Grated

Directions:

1. Get out a large pot of water and soak the rice noodles in it. Press your tofu to get out the excess liquid. Get out a nonstick pan and heat it over medium-high heat. Add in the tofu, searing for three minutes per side.
2. Whisk all ingredients for the tofu in a bowl, stirring in the tofu, and mixing well to marinate.
3. Separately mix your Thai sauce in a bowl, adding the tofu in.
4. Get a wok and put it over medium heat, adding in a teaspoon of oil.
5. Toss in the carrots, onion, red pepper, and chili. Cook for three minutes.
6. Transfer the vegetables to the tofu bowl and add in more oil. Stir the drained noodles in, and then cook for an additional minute.
7. Transfer the noodles to your tofu, and toss before serving warm. Garnish with cilantro and peanuts.

QUINOA CRANBERRY SALAD

Serves: 4

Time: 40 Minutes

Ingredients:

- 1 Cup Dry Quinoa
- 1 ½ Cups Water
- ½ cup Cranberries, Dried
- 4 Tablespoon Cilantro, Fresh & Chopped
- 1 Lime, Juiced
- 1 ½ Teaspoon Curry Powder
- 1/8 Teaspoon Cumin
- ¼ Cup Green Onion, Chopped
- ½ Cup Bell Pepper, Diced
- 1/3 Cup Toasted Almonds, Sliced
- ½ Carrots, Shredded
- 4 Tablespoons Pepitas
- Sea Salt & Black Pepper to Taste
- Olive Oil for Drizzling
- Lime Wedges to Garnish

Directions:

1. Rinse your quinoa and then throw it in a saucepan over medium heat. Cook for five minutes before adding the water.
2. Bring it to a boil before reducing your pot to a simmer. Cover and cook for thirteen minutes.
3. Toss all remaining ingredients into a salad bowl and mix with quinoa. Serve fresh.

EGGPLANT PASTA

Serves: 4

Time: 30 Minutes

Ingredients:

- 12 Ounces Dry Pasta
- 2 Cups Cremini Mushrooms, Sliced
- ½ Eggplant, Small & Cubed
- 1 ½ Cups Marinara Sauce, Preferably Vegan
- 2 Cups Water
- Sea Salt & Black Pepper to Taste
- 3 Tablespoons Olive Oil
- Basil, Fresh to Garnish

Directions:

1. Put your eggplant in a colander before sprinkling with salt. They will drain as it rests for half an hour. Rinse thoroughly after the thirty-minute mark.
2. Put a saucepan over medium-high heat with your eggplant, olive oil, ½ teaspoon of salt, and a third of your minced garlic. Stir and then cook for an additional six minutes. It should be golden brown and then add n the mushrooms. Sauté for two minutes before putting it in a bowl.
3. Cook your pasta according to package instructions and drain. Add in the marinara sauce and garlic into the saucepan with your pasta. Season with salt and pepper as necessary.
4. Toss in the eggplant and garnish with basil.

CREAM OF BROCCOLI SOUP

Serves: 6

Time: 25 Minutes

Ingredients:

- 2 Celery Stalks, Diced
- ¼ Teaspoon Thyme
- 1 Carrot, Peeled & Diced
- 2 Broccoli Heads, Chopped
- 2 Bay Leaves
- 1 Can Cannellini Beans
- 4 Cups Vegetable Broth
- 2 Cups Water
- 2 Tablespoons Nutritional Yeast
- 1 Packet Vegetable Powder

Directions:

1. **Get out a pot and add the carrot, celery, and thyme.**
2. Cover and cook for five minutes using medium heat.
3. Pour in a dash of water, then take it off of the heat. Chop the florets and stalks again after peeling. Add the stock, water, bay leaf, beans, broccoli to your carrot mixture.
4. Cover the soup, and bring it all to a boil.
5. Allow it to simmer for ten minutes, and then discard the bay leaf before taking it off of the heat.
6. Stir in the vegetable powder and nutritional powder. Blend using an immersion blender before serving.

RED LENTIL PASTA

Serves: 6

Time: 40 Minutes

Ingredients:

- 1 Tablespoon Oregano
- 1 Tablespoon Basil
- 6 Cloves Garlic, Minced
- 1 Sweet Onion, Chopped
- ¼ Cup Olive Oil
- 2 Teaspoons Turmeric
- Salt & Pepper to Taste
- 28 Ounces Fire Roasted Tomatoes
- ½ Cup Sundried Tomatoes, Oil Packed & Chopped
- 8 Ounces Red Lentil Pasta
- 1 Tablespoon Apple Cider Vinegar
- 2 Handfuls Baby Spinach, Large

Directions:

1. Get out a large pot and heat the oil over medium heat. Add your onion and cook for ten minutes.
2. Stir in the turmeric, oregano, salt, pepper, basil, and garlic, cooking for another minute. Add in the tomatoes with the juices, sundried tomatoes, and vinegar. Cook for fifteen minutes, and then use an immersion blender. Toss the spinach into your sauce, and cook for another five minutes. Boil your pasta according to the box, and serve with the spinach mixture and garnish as desired.

WHITE WINE PASTA

Serves: 4

Time: 30 Minutes

Ingredients:

Brussels:

- 16 Ounce Brussels Sprouts, Halved
- 2 Tablespoons Olive Oil
- Sea Salt & Black Pepper to Taste

Pasta:

- 4 Cloves Garlic, Chopped
- 3 Tablespoons Olive Oil
- 1/3 Cup Dry White Wine
- 4 Tablespoons Arrowroot Starch
- 1 ¾ Cup Almond Milk
- 4 Tablespoons Nutritional Yeast
- Sea Salt & Black Pepper to Taste
- 10 Ounces Vegan Pasta
- ¼ Cup Parmesan Cheese

Serving:

- Simple Greens
- Garlic Bread

Directions:

1. Heat the oven to 400, and then get a baking tray out. Spread the sprouts out, and then add the oil. Season with salt and pepper before tossing.

2. Boil the pasta al dente and then drain.
3. Heat a skillet using medium heat. Add the oil. Once it shimmers, add the garlic. Cook for an additional three minutes.
4. Stir the wine in to deglaze and then cook for an additional two minutes.
5. Whisk the almond milk and arrowroot powder, and then blend with the cheese in a food processor. Season with salt and pepper if desired.
6. Het the almond milk sauce in your skillet until it bubbles. Bake your sprouts for fifteen minutes, and then toss in the drained pasta, cheese sauce and sprouts together in a bowl before serving.

TART CABBAGE SOUP

Serves: 4

Time: 1 Hour 15 Minutes

Ingredients:

Marinade:

- 1 Tablespoon Tamari, Low Salt
- ¼ Teaspoon Liquid Smoke
- ½ Block Tofu, Firm, Diced & Drained

Soup:

- 2 Tablespoons Balsamic Vinegar
- 2 Teaspoons Garlic, Minced
- 1 Cup Leek, Chopped
- 6 Baby Bella Mushrooms, Fresh & Sliced
- 3 Cups Purple Cabbage, Chopped
- ½ Cup Bell Pepper, Chopped
- ½ Cup Sauerkraut
- 1 Teaspoon Caraway Seeds
- 2 Teaspoons Tamari, Low Salt
- 7 Cups Vegetable Broth
- 1 Tablespoon Sriracha Sauce
- 1 Tablespoon Lime Juice, Fresh

Directions:

1. Start by turning the oven to 400. Prepare your marinade and then marinate the tofu. Allow the tofu to marinate for fifteen minutes.
2. Place this tofu on a baking tray afterward, and bake for twelve minutes.

3. Get out a large pot and put it over medium heat. Add your leeks and a tablespoon of water. Stir well before cooking for five minutes. Toss in your chopped mushrooms before adding your garlic.
4. Stir well before cooking for another five minutes. Add in the vinegar. Use this to deglaze your pot.
5. Toss the sauerkraut with the juice it comes in. Add the cabbage, broth, bell pepper, hot sauce, lime juice, tamari, and caraway seeds.
6. Bring it all to a boil and then reduce it to a simmer.
7. Cook for twenty-five minutes. During this time, you'll need to stir occasionally. Stir in your tofu, and adjust seasonings if needed.

PARSNIP & MATZO SOUP

Serves: 4

Time: 1 Hour 25 Minutes

Ingredients:

Balls:

- 1 Teaspoon Garlic Powder
- 2 Teaspoons Onion Powder
- 1 ½ Cups Flour
- 1 ½ Cups Quinoa Flakes
- ¼ Teaspoon Sea Salt
- 2 Cups Water, Boiling
- 6 Tablespoons Pumpkin Puree

Soup:

- ¼ Cup Coconut Aminos
- 1 Yellow Onion, Chopped
- Black Pepper to Taste
- 5 Carrots, Peeled & Sliced
- 3 Celery Stalks, Diced
- 2 Parsnips, Sliced & Peeled
- 8 Cups Vegetable Broth
- 1 Cup Parsley, Fresh & Chopped
- 3 Tablespoons Dill, Fresh & Chopped to Garnish

Directions:

1. Heat the oven to 300, and then get a fifteen by thirteen tray. Line it with parchment paper.

2. Prepare your balls by mixing all of its ingredients in a bowl and roll into balls. Arrange them on your baking sheet. This should bake about thirty balls.

3. Bake for twenty minutes, but flip at the ten-minute mark. Allow the dish to cool for an additional ten minutes.

4. Make your soup by adding in your ingredients and bringing it to a boil in a large pot. Simmer for twenty minutes. Add in the balls, and cook for another thirty-five minutes. Garnish with dill before serving.

PESTO QUINOA

Serves: 1

Time: 25 Minutes

Ingredients:

- 1 Teaspoon Olive Oil
- 1 Cup Onion, Chopped
- 1 Clove Garlic, Minced
- 1 Cup Zucchini, Chopped
- Pinch Sea Salt
- 1 Tomato, Chopped
- 2 Tablespoons Sun-Dried Tomatoes, Chopped
- 3 Tablespoons Basil Pesto
- 2 Cups Quinoa, Cooked
- 1 Tablespoon Nutritional Yeast

Directions:

1. Heat the oil in a skillet over medium-high heat. Sauté the onion and cook for five minutes.
2. Add the garlic and cook until your onion has softened. Add in the salt and zucchini.
3. Add five minutes and then turn off the heat. Add in your sun-dried tomatoes and mix to combine. Toss in your pesto and then toss the vegetables to coat. Layer your spinach in a bowl and then quinoa. Top with your zucchini mixture, and sprinkle with nutritional yeast.

WALNUT & ORANGE PASTA

Serves: 3

Time: 40 Minutes

Ingredients:

- ½ Spaghetti Squash (or 7 Ounces Whole Grain Pasta
- 1 Orange, Juiced & Zested
- 2 Tablespoons Olive Oil
- 1 Clove Garlic, Pressed
- Sea Salt to Taste
- 3 Tablespoons Parsley, Fresh & Chopped Fine
- 10 Olives, Pitted & Chopped
- ¼ Cup Walnuts, Chopped
- 3 Tablespoons Nutritional Yeast

Directions:

1. To cook your spaghetti squash boil until soft, which will take about fifteen to twenty minutes. Scoop the flesh out of the skin, and then drain it. If using whole grain pasta, cook according to package instructions and drain well.
2. Get out a large bowl and mix your orange juice, orange zest, and a little olive oil. You'll want a ratio of half of your orange juice. Add in the pressed garlic and a dash of salt. Stir well. Add in your noodles and dress well.
3. Serve topped with parsley, chopped olives, nutritional yeast, and walnuts.

KALE & QUINOA SALAD

Serves: 4

Time: 55 Minutes

Ingredients:

Vegetables:

- 4 Carrots, Chopped & Large
- 1 Beet, Sliced Thin
- 2 Tablespoons Water
- Dash Sea Salt
- ½ Teaspoon Curry Powder

Quinoa:

- 1 ½ Cups Water
- ¾ Cup Quinoa, Rinsed Well

Dressing:

- 1/3 Cup Tahini
- 3 Tablespoons Lemon Juice, Fresh
- 2 Tablespoons Maple Syrup
- Pinch Sea Salt
- ¼ Cup Water

Salad:

- 8 Cups Kale, Chopped
- ½ Cup Cherry Tomatoes, Chopped
- 1 Avocado, Cubed
- ½ Cup Sprouts

- ¼ Cup Hemp Seeds

Directions:

1. Add your quinoa to a pot after it's been rinsed and then place it over medium heat. Stir and cook for two minutes before adding your water. Bring it to a boil, and then reduce it to a simmer.
2. Cook for an additional twenty minutes more. The quinoa should have absorbed all of the water.
3. Preheat your oven to 375. Put your carrots and beats spread out on a baking sheet. Drizzle your oil over them and then season. Toss to coat. Roast for an additional twenty minutes.
4. Prepare your dressing by mixing all ingredients.
5. Put your kale on a serving platter, topping with tomatoes, avocado, vegetables, quinoa, and additional toppings.

DINNER RECIPES

FUNG TOFU

Serves: 4

Time: 25 Minutes

Ingredients:

- ¼ Cup Soy Sauce
- ½ Cup Black Vinegar
- 1 Tablespoon Sesame Oil
- 2 Inches Ginger, Fresh, Peeled & Minced
- ¼ Cup Maple Syrup
- 3 Cloves Garlic, Minced
- 2 Blocks Tofu, Firm, Pressed & Sliced into 4 Slices
- 1 Tablespoon Sesame Seeds

Directions:

1. Mix your black vinegar, ginger, garlic, soy sauce, sesame oil, and maple syrup in a bowl. Toss in the tofu to coat, and then put the slices on a baking sheet to marinate for an hour.
2. Heat your grill to medium-high heat and grill for three minutes per side. Garnish using sesame seeds.

COCONUT CURRY NOODLES

Serves: 4

Time: 40 Minutes

Ingredients:

- ½ Tablespoon Olive
- 4 Cloves Garlic, Minced
- 2 Tablespoons Lemongrass, Minced
- 2 Tablespoons Red Curry Paste
- 1 Tablespoon Ginger, Fresh & created
- 1 Tablespoon Brown Sugar
- 2 Tablespoons Soy Sauce
- 2 Tablespoons Lime Juice, Fresh
- 1 Tablespoon Hot Chili Paste
- 12 Ounces Linguine
- 2 Cups Broccoli Florets
- 1 Cup Carrots, Shredded
- 1 Cup Edamame, Shelled
- 1 Red Bell Pepper, Sliced

Directions:

1. Get out a large pot and fill it with water. Salt it before bringing it to a boil using high heat.
2. Add in the pasta and cook to an al dente texture. Rinse under cold water to stop the cooking.
3. Get out a saucepan and place it over medium heat, heating your oil.
4. Throw in the garlic, lemongrass, and ginger. Cook for another half a minute.
5. Add in soy sauce, coconut milk, curry paste, brown sugar, chili paste, and lime juice. Stir in your curry mixture, cooking for ten minutes until it thickens.
6. Toss in the broccoli, edamame, bell pepper, carrots, and cooked pasta. Mix well before serving warm.

MUSHROOM & BEAN SOUP

Serves: 4

Time: 45 Minutes

Ingredients:

- 1 Tablespoon Olive Oil
- 16 Ounces Bella Mushrooms, Sliced
- ½ Red Onion, Chopped
- 3 Cloves Garlic, Minced
- 15 Ounces White Beans, Canned & Drained
- 1 Tablespoon Italian Seasoning, Dried
- 3 Cups Vegetable Broth
- 1 Teaspoon Rosemary, Fresh or Dried
- Pinch Hot Red Pepper Flakes
- Sea Salt & Black Pepper to Taste

Directions:

1. Get out a medium saucepan over medium heat. Heat your olive oil and add in your garlic and onions. Cook for two or three minutes or until golden brown. Add in your spices, salt, pepper, mushrooms and white beans now.
2. Cook for an additional five minutes and then add in your broth. Allow it to come to a boil. Stir in the chili flakes, reducing your heat to a simmer.
3. Allow your soup to cook for another half hour.
4. Puree with an immersion blender and serve garnished with hemp seeds, scallions, olive oil, or mushrooms as desired.

YELLOW WILD RICE SOUP

Serves: 6

Time: 1 Hour 15 Minutes

Ingredients:

- 4 Cups Vegetable Broth
- 3 Cups Water
- 15 Ounces Chickpeas, Canned
- 1 Cup Green Beans, Frozen
- 14.5 Ounces Coconut Milk, Full Fat
- Sea Salt & Black Pepper to Taste
- ½ Teaspoon Ground Ginger
- ½ Teaspoon Cumin
- 1 Teaspoon Turmeric
- ½ Teaspoon Curry Powder
- 1 Tablespoon Tomato Paste
- 1 Cup Wild Rice
- 4 Cloves Garlic, Grated
- 1 ½ Cups Mushrooms, Chopped
- ½ Cup Carrots, Chopped
- 1 Cup White Onions, Chopped
- 1 Tablespoon Coconut Oil

Directions:

1. Get out a stockpot and place it over medium heat. Add in your coconut oil and add in the onions and carrots. Sauté until soft.
2. Stir in the mushrooms and garlic cooking for three minutes.
3. Add in the spices, wild rice, tomato paste, and liquids.
4. Once it boils, you can reduce it to a simmer and allow it to simmer for an hour. Add in the green beans and chickpeas and then serve warm.

WILD RICE LEMON SOUP

Serves: 6

Time: 1 Hour 5 Minutes

Ingredients:

- 1 Cup Carrots, Chopped
- ½ Cup White Onion
- 1 Tablespoon Olive Oil
- 1Cup Celery, Sliced
- 6 Cloves Garlic, Minced
- 1 Tablespoon Lemon Zest
- Sea Salt & Black Pepper to Taste
- 1 Tablespoon Italian Seasoning
- ½ Cup Wild Rice
- 4 Cups Vegetable Broth
- 1 Cup Almond Milk
- ¼ Cup Lemon Juice, Fresh
- 1 Cup Spinach, Fresh

Directions:

1. Get out a Dutch oven and add your oil to it. Place it over medium heat, and then toss in the carrots, garlic, celery, and onion. Cook for five minutes.
2. Stir in your zest and the remaining seasoning, cooking for three minutes. Add in the wild rice and vegetable broth.
3. Allow it to come to a boil and then reduce the heat to a simmer.
4. Cover and allow it to cook for forty minutes.
5. Add the spinach, milk, and lemon juice.
6. Leave it covered for five minutes and allow it to serve warm.

CARROT & TURMERIC SOUP

Serves: 4

Time: 1 Hour

Ingredients:

- 1 Tablespoon Olive Oil
- 1 Cup Fennel, Chopped
- 1 Leek, Sliced Thin
- 3 Cups Carrots, Chopped
- 1 Cup Butternut Squash, Chopped
- 3 Cloves Garlic, Minced
- 1 Tablespoon Ginger, Grated
- 1 Tablespoon Turmeric Powder
- Sea Salt & Black Pepper to Taste
- 3 Cups Vegetable Broth
- 14.5 Ounces Coconut Milk, Canned

Directions:

1. Get out a Dutch oven and place it over medium heat to heat your olive oil.
2. Stir in your fennel, carrots, leeks, and squash. Cook for five minutes. Toss your garlic, ginger, salt, pepper, and turmeric in next. Stir and cook for another two minutes. Pour in your broth and coconut milk next.
3. Once it comes to a boil, cover it and reduce it to a simmer. Allow it to simmer for twenty minutes.
4. Once it's cooked, puree it using an immersion blender and garnish with coconut yogurt.

BLACKEYE PEA BURRITOS

Serves: 6

Time: 50 Minutes

Ingredients:

- 1 Teaspoon Olive Oil
- 1 Red Onion, Diced
- 2 Cloves Garlic, Minced
- 1 Zucchini, Chopped
- 1 Bell Pepper, Seeded & Diced
- 1 Tomato, Diced
- 2 Teaspoons Chili Powder
- Sea Salt to Taste
- 14 Ounces Blackeye Peas, Rinsed & Drained
- 6 Tortillas, Whole Grain

Directions:

1. Start by turning your oven to 325, and then get out a skillet. Put it over medium heat, and add in the oil and onion. Cook for five minutes before adding the garlic. Cook for less than a minute more. Add the bell pepper and tomato, and cook for two to three more minutes.
2. When your tomato is warmed, add in your slat, blackeye peas, and chili powder. Stir well.
3. Place in the center of tortillas and roll like a burrito.
4. Place these burritos in a baking dish and pour in the vegetable juice. Continue cooking for twenty to thirty minutes.

PLANT-BASED SHEPARD'S PIE

Serves: 6

Time: 1 Hour

Ingredients:

- 1 Cup Lentils
- 6 Potatoes, Peeled
- ¼ Cup Almond Milk
- 1 Tablespoon Coconut Oil
- 1 Yellow Onion, Diced
- 1 Teaspoon Olive Oil
- 2 Carrots, Diced
- ½ Cup Peas, Fresh or Frozen
- 2 Tablespoons Red Wine
- 1 Tablespoon Thyme, Fresh & Chopped
- 2 Teaspoons Sea Salt
- Black Pepper to Taste
- 2 Tablespoons Whole Grain Flour
- ½ Cup Water

Directions:

1. Place your lentils in a pot with three cups of water. Bring it to a boil before allowing it to simmer for thirty minutes or until soft.

2. During this time, cut your potatoes into chunks and place them in a large pot. Fill with water until the potatoes are covered well. Add a little salt and bring your potatoes to a boil for twenty minutes. They should soften. When cooked, drain and leave only a half a cup of cooking liquid with them. Mash until smooth, only adding liquid if necessary. Add nondairy milk if desired and season with salt.

3. Heat the oven to 350, and then drain your lentils. Transfer them to a nine-inch pie pan. You can also use a baking dish.
4. Take the pot your cooked lentils in now that it's empty and cook your onion and olive oil. Cook your lentils for five minutes more before throwing your carrots in. Cook another five minutes and then add in the peas, wine, and thyme. Add this to the lentils, season with salt, pepper, and flour. Stir well and then add water to dissolve the flour.
5. Spread your mashed potatoes over the lentils, baking for twenty to thirty minutes. It should be golden brown.

PAD THAI BOWL

Serves: 2

Time: 20 Minutes

Ingredients:

- ¼ Cup Peanut Sauce
- ¼ Cup Cilantro, Fresh & Chopped Fine
- 2 Tablespoons Roasted Peanuts, Chopped
- Fresh Lime Wedges to Garnish
- 1 Cup Bean Sprouts
- 2-3 Tablespoons Mint, Fresh & Chopped Fine
- 2 Scallions, Finely Chopped
- 1 Red Bell Pepper, Seeded & Sliced Thin
- 1 Cup Napa Cabbage, Sliced Thin
- 2 Carrots, Peeled & Julienned
- 1 Teaspoon Olive Oil
- 7 Ounces Brown Rice Noodles

Directions:

1. Place your rice noodles in a large bowl and cover with boiling water. Allow it to sit for ten minutes. The noodles should soften. Rinse, drain, and then allow them to cool.
2. Heat a large skillet over medium-high heat with the oil in it. sauté your cabbage, carrots, and bell pepper for seven to eight minutes. Toss in your mint, bean sprouts, and scallions. Cook the dish for two more minutes before taking it off of the heat.
3. Toss the noodles in, and then add in the peanut sauce.
4. Transfer bowls and then sprinkle with peanuts and cilantro to serve with lime wedges.

GINGER SOBA NOODLE BOWL

Serves: 2

Time: 25 Minutes

Ingredients:

Bowl:

- 7 Ounces Soba Noodles
- 1 Bell Pepper, Sliced Thin
- 1 Carrot, Peeled & Julienned
- 1 Cup Snow peas, Trimmed
- 2 Tablespoons Scallions, Chopped
- 1 Cup Kale, Chopped
- 1 Avocado, Sliced Thin
- 2 Tablespoons Cashews, Chopped

Dressing:

- 1 Tablespoon Ginger, Fresh & Grated
- 2 Tablespoons Cashew Butter
- 2 Tablespoons Rice Vinegar
- 2 Tablespoons Tamari
- 1 Teaspoon Sesame Oil, Toasted
- 2-3 Tablespoons Water

Directions:

1. Get a medium pot of water boiling and add the noodles in. Make sure it's a low boil, and turn down the heat if necessary. Cook for six to seven minutes, and stir every few minutes to prevent sticking. Drain and rinse with cold water to stop the cooking.
2. Chop your vegetables and place them in a skillet over medium-high heat until tender.

3. Make your dressing by squeezing your grated ginger to get the juice, and then whisk all ingredients together. Puree in a blender and set it to the side.

4. Arrange your bowl with kale or spinach on the bottom, then the noodles, drizzle with tamari sauce. Add the vegetable sand dressing next. Top with avocado and chopped cashews before serving.

BIBIMBAP BOWL

Serves: 1

Time: 30 Minutes

Ingredients:

- ½ Cup Bean Sprouts
- 3 Tablespoons Hot Pepper Paste
- 1 Tablespoon Toasted Sesame Seeds
- 1 Scallion, Chopped
- ½ Cup Spinach, Fresh & Chopped
- ½ Cup Asparagus, Chopped into 2 Inch Pieces
- 2 Cloves Garlic, Minced & Divided
- Pinch Sea Salt
- 1 Carrot, Peeled & Julienned
- 1 Teaspoon Olive Oil
- ¾ Cup Brown Rice, Cooked
- 1 Tablespoon + 2 Teaspoons Toasted Sesame Oil, Divided
- 2 Tablespoons Tamari
- ½ Cup Chickpeas, Cooked

Directions:

1. Get out a small bowl and toss the chickpeas with a teaspoon of sesame oil and a tablespoon of tamari. Allow your chickpeas to marinate.
2. Place the rice in a serving bowl.
3. Heat your oil in a skillet over medium heat, and then sauté your carrot and some clove. Add a dash of salt and cook for about five minutes. Place them on top of the rice.

4. Sauté your asparagus, adding more oil only if necessary. Drizzle with the remaining tablespoon of tamari and teaspoon of sesame oil. Add the spinach and carrots into the bowl on the other side of the asparagus.

5. Sauté your bean sprouts lightly or serve them raw. This is according to your preference.

6. Put the marinated chickpeas in the bowl.

7. Get out another small bowl and mix your hot pepper paste with a tablespoon of sesame oil.

8. Place this in the middle of the bowl and garnish with scallions and sesame seeds.

SESAME STIR FRY

Serves: 4

Time: 30 Minutes

Ingredients:

- 2 Cups Water
- 1 Cup Quinoa
- Pinch Sea Salt
- 1 Head Broccoli
- 2 Teaspoons Sesame Oil
- 1 Cup Snow Peas, Trimmed
- 1 Cup Edamame, Frozen & Shelled
- 2 Cups Swiss Chard, Chopped
- 2 Scallions, Chopped
- 2 Tablespoons Water
- 1 Tablespoon Tamari
- 1 Teaspoon Toasted Sesame Oil
- 2 Tablespoons Sesame Seeds

Directions:

1. Place your water, salt, and quinoa in a pot and then bring it to a boil. Reduce to low and allow it to simmer for twenty minutes. When your quinoa is cooked, do not fluff or stir.
2. Cut your broccoli into florets and then chop your stem into small pieces.
3. Put a skillet over high heat and sauté your broccoli and sesame oil with a pinch of salt. Make sure it doesn't burn and drizzle more oil as needed. Add the rest of the vegetables and sauté. Your swiss chard should only be in there long enough for it to wilt. Add two tablespoons of hot water if needed.
4. Dress with tamari and sesame oil and remove from heat. Serve on top of quinoa.

SUNDAY ROAST

Serves: 8

Time: 4-6 Hours

Ingredients:

- 6 White Potatoes, Cubed
- 6 Carrots, Sliced into ½ Inch Rounds
- 3 Sweet Onions, Sliced into ½ Inch Cubes
- 12 Ounces Green Beans, Fresh
- 8 Ounces Mushrooms, Sliced
- 4 Cups Vegetable Broth
- 1 Teaspoon Garlic Powder
- 1 Teaspoon Onion Powder
- 1 Teaspoon Black Pepper

Directions:

1. Throw everything into a slow cooker, and mix well.
2. Cook for four to six hours on high, and the dish will be done. You could also cook for six to eight hours on low. Stir well before serving.

TOFU BOWL

Serves: 4

Time: 55 Minutes

Ingredients:

Tofu:

- ¼ Cup Whole Wheat Flour
- 1 Teaspoon Onion Powder
- 1 Teaspoon Garlic Powder
- ½ Teaspoon Black Pepper
- 14 Ounces Firm Tofu, Drained & Cubed

Glaze:

- 1 Tablespoon Cornstarch
- ½ Cup Orange Juice, Pulp Free
- 1 Tablespoon Rice Vinegar
- 1 Tablespoon Maple Syrup
- ½ Teaspoon Onion Powder
- ½ Teaspoon Garlic Powder
- 6 Cups Brown Rice, Cooked to Serve

Directions:

1. Heat your oven to 400 and get a baking sheet lined with parchment paper. Get a bowl out and whisk the garlic, onion, pepper, and flour. Toss in the tofu, making sure it's coated.
2. Place this on a baking sheet, baking for forty minutes and turning twenty minutes in.

3. Get out a saucepan while your tofu is baking and combine the cornstarch, rice vinegar, orange juice, maple syrup, garlic powder, and onion powder. Bring it to a boil using medium-high heat. Reduce to low, and allow it to simmer for ten minutes.
4. Mix the glaze with the tofu and serve over rice.

MANGO CHICKPEA CURRY

Serves: 6

Time: 20 Minutes

Ingredients:

- 3 Cups Chickpeas, Cooked
- 2 Cups Mango Chunks, Fresh
- 2 Cups Almond Milk
- 2 Tablespoons Maple Syrup
- 1 Tablespoon Curry Powder
- 1 Teaspoon Ground Coriander
- 1 Tablespoon ground Ginger
- 1 Teaspoon Garlic Powder
- 1 Teaspoon Onion Powder
- 1/8 Teaspoon Ground Cinnamon

Directions:

1. Get out a Dutch oven and heat it over medium heat.
2. Combine the mango, milk, chickpeas, maple syrup, ginger, curry powder, garlic powder, onion powder, cinnamon, and coriander. Cover, cooking for ten minutes, but stir halfway through.
3. Uncover, and cook for five minutes more.

STUFFED SOUTHWEST PEPPERS

Serves: 4

Time: 40 Minutes

Ingredients:

- 4 Bell Peppers
- 3 Cups Brown Rice, Cooked
- 1 Cup Black Beans, Cooked
- 1 Cup Corn, Fresh or Frozen
- 1 Cup Vegetable Broth
- 2 Tablespoons Chili Powder
- 2 Tablespoons Tomato Paste
- 1 Teaspoon Ground Cumin

Directions:

1. Heat the oven to 375, and then slice the top off of your bell peppers and seed them.
2. Get out a bowl and mix your corn, beans, broth, rice, tomato paste, cumin, and chili powder. Mix well and then spoon a quarter of your rice mixture into each pepper. Stand them in a baking dish upright, and bake for an hour.

SIDE DISH RECIPES

CARROT & CHICKPEA SALAD

Serves: 8

Time: 20 Minutes

Ingredients:

- Large Handful Lettuce
- 1 Teaspoon Apple Cider Vinegar
- ½ Cup Vegan Cream
- Sea Salt & Black Pepper to Taste
- ½ Teaspoon Oregano
- 1 Onion, Small
- 3 Pickles
- 14 Ounces Chickpeas, Canned

Carrots:

- 8 Carrots, Large
- 1 Tablespoon Oil
- 1 ½ Teaspoons Sea Salt, Fine
- 1 Teaspoon Oregano
- 1 Teaspoon Thyme
- 2 Teaspoons Paprika Powder
- 1 ½ Tablespoon Soy Sauce
- ½ Cup Water

Directions:

1. Toss in all of the ingredients for your carrot in a bowl.
2. Thread them on sticks and place them on a plate until your grill is ready. Heat the grill to high heat, and then grill for two minutes per side.
3. Toss all ingredients for your salad together, and top with carrots before serving warm. Alternatively, you can slice the carrots.

PLANTAIN CHIPS

Serves: 4

Time: 25 Minutes

Ingredients:

- ¼ Teaspoon Cumin
- ½ Teaspoon Smoked Paprika
- 1 Green Plantain, Sliced

Directions:

1. Start by turning your grill to medium heat and then get out an aluminum sheet. Grease using cooking spray, and then spread out the plantain slices. Drizzle with paprika and cumin. Place this sheet on the grill.
2. Cover your grill and cook for seven minutes. Flip the plantain slices using a tong, and then cover again.
3. Cook for an additional seven minutes before serving the dish warm.

STUFFED PORTOBELLO

Serves: 6

Time: 1 Hour 30 Minutes

Ingredients:

- ½ Cup Mint, Fresh
- ½ Cup Basil, Fresh
- 1 Cup Wild Rice
- ½ Cup Parsley, Fresh
- 1 Tablespoon Olive Oil
- 1 Tablespoon Nutritional Yeast
- 1 Lemon, Zested
- ½ Lemon, Juiced
- 1 Teaspoon Honey, Raw
- ¾ Cup Pecans
- 6 Portobello Mushrooms, Large
- Coconut Oil to Grease
- Sea Salt & Black Pepper to Taste

Directions:

1. Get a saucepan and place three cups of water in with your wild rice. Season with sea salt, and then place the lid on.
2. Cook your rice using a simmer for fifty minutes.
3. Drain the rice, and then spread your pecans on a baking sheet. Turn the oven to 375, and then roast for eight minutes. Shake once during this time.
4. Chop your pecans, and then set the chopped pecans to the side.
5. Blend your basil, olive oil, parsley, mint, lemon juice, zest, nutritional yeast, salt, and honey in a blender.

6. Clean your mushrooms before brushing them down with coconut oil. Drizzle your mushrooms with salt and pepper, and then heat the grill to medium-high heat. Grill your mushrooms for six minutes per side, and then stuff each mushroom with pesto, wild rice, and your pecans. Garnish with lemon zest before serving.

ROASTED CHICKPEAS

Serves: 4

Time: 30 Minutes

Ingredients:

- 14 Ounces Chickpeas, Rinsed & Drained
- 2 Tablespoons Tamari
- 1 Tablespoon Nutritional Yeast
- 1 Teaspoon Onion Powder
- ½ Teaspoon Garlic Powder
- 1 Teaspoon Smoked Paprika

Directions:

1. Turn the oven to 400 and then add all ingredients together. Mix well and then spread them out on a baking dish. Bake for twenty minutes. Toss halfway through. Bake for an additional five if not golden.

PESTO POTATOES

Serves: 4

Time: 30 Minutes

Ingredients:

- 2 Teaspoons Olive Oil
- 8 Cloves Garlic, Peeled
- 8 Potatoes, Small & Peeled
- Sea Salt to Taste
- ¼ Cup Basil Pesto

Directions:

1. Start by heating your oven to 350, and then chop the potatoes. Get out a bowl and toss everything together.
2. Get out a baking dish and then throw in the mixture. Bake your potato mixture for twenty-five minutes.
3. Toss in pesto before serving.

SWEET POTATO CASSEROLE

Serves: 6

Time: 30 Minutes

Ingredients:

- 1 Tablespoon Sage
- 1 Teaspoon Thyme
- 1 Teaspoon Rosemary
- ½ Cup Vegetable Broth
- 8 Sweet Potatoes, Cooked

Directions:

1. Heat the oven to 375, and then skin the sweet potatoes. Put them in the dish, and mash. Stir in all remaining ingredients.
2. Bake your dish for a half-hour before serving.

EASY COLLARD GREENS

Serves: 4

Time: 25 Minutes

Ingredients:

- Black Pepper to Taste
- ½ Teaspoon Onion Powder
- ½ Teaspoon Garlic Powder
- 1 Cup Vegetable Broth
- 1 ½ lb. Collard Greens

Directions:

1. Remove the hard stems, and chop your leaves roughly. Get out a saucepan and mix your garlic powder, onion powder, pepper, and vegetable broth. Bring the mix to a boil using medium-high heat. Add in the greens, and lower the heat to a simmer.
2. Cover the dish and cook for twenty minutes. Stir every five to six minutes. Serve warm.

SESAME FRIES

Serves: 4

Time: 35 Minutes

Ingredients:

- 1 lb. Gold Potatoes, Unpeeled & Sliced into Wedges
- 2 Tablespoons Sesame Seeds
- 1 Tablespoon Avocado Oil
- 1 Tablespoon Potato Starch
- 1 Tablespoon Nutritional Yeast
- Sea Salt & Black Pepper to Taste

Directions:

1. Heat your oven to 425, and then get out a baking tray. Line with parchment paper, and put your potatoes onto the tray. Toss with remaining ingredients.
2. Bake for twenty-five minutes, tossing halfway through.

VEGETABLE STIR FRY

Serves: 10

Time: 20 Minutes

Ingredients:

- 1 Tablespoon Oil
- 1 Onion, Sliced
- 1 Cup Carrots, Sliced
- 2 Cups Broccoli Florets
- 2 Cups Sugar Snap Peas
- 1 Large Red Bell Pepper, Chopped into Strips
- 1 Tablespoon Soy Sauce, Reduced Sodium
- 1 Teaspoon Garlic Powder
- 1 Teaspoon Ginger
- 2 Teaspoons Sesame Seeds, Toasted

Directions:

1. Get out a deep skillet over medium-high heat to heat the oil. Toss in the onions and carrots, cooking for two minutes. Stir in the rest of the ingredients, cooking for an additional seven minutes.
2. Add the soy sauce, ginger, and garlic. Garnish with sesame seeds and serve warm.

VEGETABLE SATAY

Serves: 4

Time: 30 Minutes

Ingredients:

- 1 Cup Vegetable Broth
- 1 Tablespoon Cornstarch
- 1 Tablespoon Soy Sauce, Low Sodium
- 1 Tablespoon Vegetable Oil
- 1 Cup Broccoli Florets
- 1 Cup Cauliflower Florets
- 1 Cup Baby Carrots
- 2 Teaspoons Ginger Root, Fresh & Grated
- 2 Stalks Celery, Sliced
- 2 Cloves Garlic, Minced
- ½ Teaspoon Sesame Seeds

Directions:

1. Mix the soy sauce, broth, and cornstarch in a bowl. It should be smooth.
2. Place a medium skillet over medium-high heat, and add in the oil.
3. Toss the vegetables in only once the oil is heated. Sauté until crisp.
4. Stir in the broth mixture. Bring it to a boil and garnish with sesame seeds.

WINTER HASH

Serves: 6

Time: 40 Minutes

Ingredients:

- 3 Tablespoons Olive Oil
- 2 Tablespoons Butter
- ½ lbs. Shitake Mushrooms, Diced
- 1 lb. Gold Potatoes, Diced
- 1 Red Bell Pepper, Diced
- 1 Small Acorn Squash, Diced
- 1 Shallot, Chopped Fine
- 2 Teaspoons Garlic Powder
- Sea Salt & Black Pepper to Taste
- 1 Cup Kale, Chopped
- 4 Sprigs Sage, Fresh

Directions:

1. Pour your butter, oil, and broth into a skillet. Cook using medium heat, and then add in the vegetables and seasoning. Do not add in your kale or sage yet.
2. Cook for twenty-five minutes while stirring occasionally. The vegetables should be tender and then add kale and sage. Cook the dish for an additional five minutes.

FRENCH POTATO SALAD

Serves: 14

Time: 25 Minutes

Ingredients:

Dressing:

- ¼ Cup Dill, Fresh & Chopped
- 3 Tablespoons Olive Oil
- 1 Tablespoon Apple Cider Vinegar
- 3 Tablespoons Red Wine Vinegar
- Sea Salt & Black Pepper to Taste
- 3 Cloves Garlic, Minced
- 2 ½ Tablespoons Spicy Brown Mustard

Potatoes & Vegetables:

- 2 lb. Baby Yellow potatoes
- Sea Salt & Black Pepper to Taste
- 1 Tablespoon Apple Cider Vinegar
- 1 Cup Green Onion, Diced
- ¼ Cup Parsley, Fresh & Chopped

Directions:

1. Wash your potatoes before chopping them into ¼ inch slices. Put the slices in a pan, preferably a saucepan, and then add the water. Add a pinch of salt.
2. Boil for fifteen minutes. Your potatoes should be soft. Drain and rinse using cold water.
3. Add the potatoes to a serving bowl, seasoning with apple cider vinegar, and then a dash of salt and pepper.
4. Whisk all remaining ingredients together in a separate bowl. Mix well before serving.

DESSERT
RECIPES

CHOCOLATE BANANA CUPCAKES

Serves: 12

Time: 45 Minutes

Ingredients:

- 3 Bananas
- 1 Cup Almond Milk
- 2 Tablespoons Almond Butter
- 1 Teaspoon Apple Cider Vinegar
- 1 Teaspoon Vanilla Extract, Pure
- 1 ¼ Cups Whole Grain Flour
- ½ Cup Rolled Oats
- ¼ Cup Coconut Sugar
- 1 Teaspoon Baking Powder
- ½ Cup Cocoa Powder, Unsweetened
- ½ Teaspoon Baking Soda
- Pinch Sea Salt
- ¼ Cup Chia Seeds
- ¼ Cup Dark Chocolate Chips

Directions:

1. Heat the oven to 350, and get out a muffin pan. Grease it. Place your almond butter, vinegar, milk, bananas, and vanilla together. Puree until smooth.
2. Place the flour, sugar, oats, baking soda, baking powder, chia seeds, cocoa powder, chocolate chips, and salt together in a bowl. Mix well.
3. Mix your wet and dry ingredients, and make sure there are no lumps.
4. Spoon into muffin cups and bake for twenty to twenty-five minutes.
5. Allow them to cool before serving. They should be moist.

COCONUT CHIA PUDDING

Serves: 4

Time: 30 Minutes

Ingredients:

- 1 Lime, Juiced & Zested
- 14 Ounces Coconut Milk, Canned
- 2 Dates
- 2 Tablespoons Chia Seeds, Ground
- 2 Teaspoons Matcha Powder

Directions:

1. Get out a blender and blend everything until smooth. Chill for twenty minutes before serving.

MANGO CREAM PIE

Serves: 8

Time: 50 Minutes

Ingredients:

Crust:

- ½ Cup Rolled Oats
- 1 Cup Cashews
- 1 Cup Dates, Pitted

Filling:

- 2 Mangos, Large, Peeled & Chopped
- ½ Cup Water
- 1 Cup Coconut Milk, Canned
- ½ Cup Coconut, Shredded & Unsweetened

Directions:

1. Get out a food processor and pulse all of your crust ingredients together. Press into an eight-inch pie pan.
2. Blend all filling ingredients. It should be thick and make sure it's smooth.
3. Pour it into the crust, and smooth out. Allow it to set in the freezer for thirty minutes.
4. Allow it to come to room temperature for ten to fifteen minutes before slicing.

AVOCADO BLUEBERRY CHEESECAKE

Serves: 8

Time: 2 Hours 20 Minutes

Ingredients:

Crust:

- 1 Cup Rolled Oats
- 1 Cup Walnuts
- 1 Teaspoon Lime Zest
- 1 Cup Soft Pitted Dates

Filling:

- 2 Tablespoons Maple Syrup
- 1 Cup Blueberries, Frozen
- 2 Avocados, Peeled & Pitted
- 2 Tablespoons Basil, Fresh & Minced Fine
- 4 Tablespoons Lime Juice

Directions:

1. Pulse all crust ingredients together in your food processor, and then press into a pie pan.
2. Blend all filling ingredients until smooth, and pour it into the crust. Smooth out and freeze for two hours before serving.

SPICE CAKE

Serves: 6

Time: 50 Minutes

Ingredients:

- 1 Sweet Potato, Cooked & Peeled
- ½ Cup Applesauce, Unsweetened
- ½ Cup Almond Milk
- ¼ Cup Maple Syrup, Pure
- 1 Teaspoon Vanilla Extract, Pure
- 2 Cups Whole Wheat Flour
- ½ Teaspoon Ground Cinnamon
- ½ Teaspoon Baking Soda
- ¼ Teaspoon Ground Ginger

Directions:

1. Turn your oven to 350, and then get a large bowl out. Mash your sweet potatoes and then mix in the vanilla, milk, and maple syrup. Mix well.
2. Stir in the baking soda, cinnamon, flour, and ginger. Mix well.
3. Pour this batter into a baking dish that's been lined with parchment paper. Bake the batter for forty-five minutes.
4. Allow it to cool before slicing to serve.

LEMON CAKE

Serves: 10

Time: 5 Hours 10 Minutes

Ingredients:

Crust:

- 1 Cup Dates, Pitted
- 2 Tablespoons Maple Syrup
- 2 ½ Cups Pecans

Filling:

- 1 Lemon, Juiced & Zested
- ¾ Cup Maple Syrup
- 1 ½ Cups Pineapple, Crushed
- 3 Cups Cauliflower Rice, Prepared
- 3 Avocados, Halved & Pitted
- ½ Teaspoon Vanilla Extract, Pure
- ½ Teaspoon Lemon Extract
- 1 Pinch Cinnamon

Topping:

- 1 Teaspoon Vanilla Extract, Pure
- 1 ½ Cups Coconut Yogurt, Plain
- 3 Tablespoons Maple Syrup

Directions:

1. Get a nine-inch springform pan out, lining it with parchment paper.

2. Put your pecans in a food processor, grinding until fine. Stir in the maple syrup and dates, blending for a minute more. Spread this into your pan to make the crust.

3. Blend your maple syrup, pineapple, lemon juice, lemon zest, cauliflower rice, and avocados in a food processor. Add in the lemon extract, cinnamon, and vanilla. Mix well.

4. Top your crust with this mixture, and freeze for five hours.

5. To make your topping whisk all ingredients together, spreading it over your prepared cake.

BUTTERSCOTCH TART

Serves: 10

Time: 50 Minutes

Ingredients:

Crust:

- ½ Cup Sugar
- ¼ Cup Coconut Oil
- 1 Teaspoon Vanilla Extract, Pure
- ½ Teaspoon Sea Salt
- 2 Cups Almond Meal Flour

Filling:

- 2/3 Cup Light Brown Sugar, Packed
- 1 Teaspoon Kosher Salt
- ½ Cup Coconut Oil
- 2/3 Cup Coconut Cream, Canned
- Flaked Sea Salt, As Needed
- 1 Green Apple, Sliced

Directions:

1. Turn the oven to 375, and then get out a bowl. Prepare your crust ingredients by mixing everything until smooth. Spread this into a tart pan that's nine inches. Spread it as evenly as possible. Freeze for ten minutes, and then bake for fifteen. It should be golden brown.
2. Prepare the filling by cooking it al in a saucepan for twenty-five minutes. It should thicken and allow it to cool. You will need to stir often to keep it from burning.
3. Add this to the tart, and then chill for two hours before serving.

EASY BROWNIES

Serves: 12

Time: 25 Minutes

Ingredients:

- 2 Tablespoons Coconut Oil, Melted
- ½ Cup Peanut Butter, Salted
- ¼ Cup Warm Water
- 2 Cups Dates, Pitted
- 1/3 Cup Dark Chocolate chips
- 1/3 Cup Cocoa Powder
- ½ Cup Raw Walnuts, Chopped

Directions:

1. Heat the oven to 350, and then get out a loaf pan. Place parchment paper in it, and then get out a food processor. Blend your dates until it's a fine mixture. Add in some hot water, and blend well until the mixture become an as smooth batter.
2. Add in the coconut oil, cacao powder, and peanut butter. Blend more, and then fold in the chocolate and walnuts. Spread this into your loaf pan.
3. Bake for fifteen minutes, and then chill before serving.

CONCLUSION

Now you know everything you need to get started on a plant-based diet. Plant-based diets are easy to follow because you aren't required to take them into your everyday life. Just keep to a plant-based diet in the kitchen and when out with friends to help you meet your weight loss as well as your health goals. Everything from delicious smoothies to exotic dinner dishes such as pad Thai can still be yours. There's no reason to give up taste for health with the plant-based diet, so there's no reason not to get started today. With a twenty-one-day meal plan, it's easier than ever.

Made in the USA
Monee, IL
02 September 2020